DENTAL HEAVEN

How to Have A Great Smile
and Healthy Mouth
Without Paying Through the Nose

By Ellen L. Hughes

Published by The McKee Company
P.O. Box 22996
Denver, CO 80222
www.themckeecompany.com

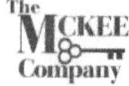

Table of Contents

I. INTRODUCTION

It was time for a visit to the dentist. I knew I would need some work done and had dental insurance to help defray the costs. Even with that cushion, the total was $945 for fillings, cleaning and a night guard. After their fourth attempt to fit the night guard I told them I would go somewhere else. I also told them that one of my teeth still needed a filling because I could feel sensation in it when I drank something cold. They informed me I would have to pay an additional $130 for the filling.

We all reach a breaking point. That was mine. I have spent my life in a dentist's office. My life in "the chair" started in first grade when I broken a tooth on the playground. A cap for a broken front tooth was the beginning of many "rinse and spit" sessions. (*A suction tube has taken the place of spraying water in the mouth and then spit out. I miss the rinse and spit.*). Next it was braces for an overbite. Then came another cap, fillings, removal of wisdom teeth, and...well you get it. I know my way around a dental office.

Through the years I have seen a change from personal, professional service to a more impersonal, assembly-line feel. The quality of service has plummeted while costs have risen drastically.

A few years ago, a friend who is a world traveler told me he always had his dental work done in Mexico. I didn't ask him details then but I decided now was the time to find out more about this option. Because in additional to needing the filling ($130) and night guard ($195), I needed a root canal ($1200 with porcelain crown).

It was time to explore other options. Finding a dentist who was qualified and capable, gave personal service and charged reasonable prices was becoming as scarce as hen's teeth.

UPDATE: I have returned to Los Algodones for more work. These new observations are also included.

The information in this book is based on personal experience, and the dental services received. No guarantees are made as to service another person may receive or fees charged.

II. PRICING

I contacted my friend, Tony, to get his dental recommendations. He gave me the name, website and e-mail of his dentist in Mexico. I checked the website and found pricing for various services. In the U.S., with my current dental insurance plan, a porcelain crown was $605; a root canal was $400, and a filling was $130, for a total of $1,135. In Mexico, the same procedures would cost a total of $420. That is a savings of $715, which more than covered the flight, hotel and rental car.

Why is dental work so much cheaper in Mexico? The reasons are many. It is cheaper to live in Mexico. Mexican dentists don't have to buy malpractice insurance and they generally don't have to track down reimbursements from insurance companies. Also, they don't have as much student debt and don't have as many regulations.

Additional Costs

Going to Mexico for dental work was starting to look like a viable option. However, there was a lot of research to be done before making a final decision, things like contacting the dentist, pricing for hotel, airfare from Denver and rental car, safety and language issues and obtaining a passport. Unless otherwise noted, the remainder of this book is research I did in preparation for my first "dental trip" to Mexico.

Second Trip

Note: Because I had such a pleasant experience on my first trip, I returned for more work in September 2014. To be fair, I gave my U.S. dentist the first opportunity. I visited them to get an estimate. They were professional, pleasant and performed a thorough examination. They were supposed to get back to me once they contacted my insurance company. They never did even though I left two messages. Their estimate (*without insurance*) was $2,210 for deep cleaning and $18,303 for work, for a total of **$20,513**. When I didn't hear back from them, I contacted the dentist in Mexico. The total for the same work was less than **$3,000**.

It wasn't even a contest. The decision had been made for me. I returned to Los Algodones in February 2015 to get one crown repaired.

III. PREPARATION FOR THE TRIP

Contacting the Dentist

I never actually spoke with the dentist that my friend recommended. (*I would recommend Skyping the doctor's office.*) We conducted all our communication via e-mail. I e-mailed him one day and received a detailed, friendly reply from him two days later. The first thing that struck me was that he said not only was Tony his patient, but he was his friend. I liked him right away.

In my e-mail I told him the work I needed done, asked how many appointments it would take for the root canal and if he wanted my X-rays. He told me to send the X-rays and said he did perform all the services I needed. Dr. C told me he would make an appointment for me on a Monday morning and be able to finish on Thursday afternoon, with 2-3 appointments in between.

We traded a few other e-mails regarding various things such as scheduling the appointment, deciding I could bring the X-rays with me instead of mailing them and hotel recommendations.

Getting A Passport

Getting into *Mexico is not a problem. To leave Mexico, you need a passport or passport card. The following rules apply for American citizens. When applying for a passport, you must apply in person if:*

> •*You are applying for your first U.S. passport*
> •*You are under age 16*
> •*Your previous U.S. passport was issued when you were under age 16*
> •*Your previous U.S. passport was lost, stolen, or damaged*
> •*Your previous U.S. passport was issued more than 15 years ago*
> •*Your name has changed since your U.S. passport was issued and you are unable to legally document your name change*

If you are renewing your passport, you may renew by mail if your current U.S. passport:

-is undamaged and can be submitted with your application
-was issued when you were age 16 or older
-was issued within the last 15 years

-was issued in your current name or you can legally document your name change

If any of the above statements do not apply to you, you must apply in person.

Processing Times

Routine Service - Normal processing time for routine service is 4-6 weeks from time of application.

Expedited Service - If you request overnight delivery and pay for shipping to and from the passport agency, you can receive your passport within 2-3 weeks.

IMPORTANT: *Please note processing times can change. For current times, visit http://www.travel.state.gov/passport and look at the left side of the page for passport information. You can also call the National*

Passport Information Center at 1-877-487-2778.

Obtaining X-Rays

By law, dentists have to give you a copy of your x-rays and all records. Some offices may charge for the copies. Some dentists will only give out records to the new dental office and not to the patient. Should that happen, you can threaten them with legal action. The law is behind you.
Ask your dentist in Mexico if they want you to send the X-rays or bring them with you. They may not even want them and prefer to make new X-rays.

Hotel/Airfare/Car Rental

You will be traveling to Yuma, Arizona. This is not your final destination. Los Algodones, Mexico is where you will go for dental work. But you will go to Yuma in order to get to Los Algodones. We will discuss the town itself a little later.

I flew into Yuma from Denver via US Airways for $212.40. You will need to check airfare from your city. At the time, I used Travelocity.com to find the best deals. The rules have changed and now it is better to book directly with the airline itself. It is best to book your flight on a Tuesday..   I have personally witnessed the prices decrease from Monday fees to what is charged on Tuesday and then increase again on Wednesday.

The terminal in Yuma is small. It has only a couple of restaurants and no shops (that I saw). According to their website, there are four automobile rental agencies, a restaurant and lounge and a game room. I rented a car from Enterprise for $161.37 for the week. I arrived on Sunday and left on Friday, so the charge was for a full week. There were many problems with the car, including a smell that wouldn't go away. I had to return it twice. Enterprise ended up reducing my rate because of these problems. I have rented from Enterprise several times and never had any problems before. I am assuming this time was an anomaly, but wanted to give full disclosure.
Next on to the lodging. I chose Motel 6 because they have always been clean and inexpensive. I figured since I was going to be sitting in a dentist's chair for most of the week, why spend a lot on a room to

sleep in? I stayed at the Motel 6 on E. 16th Street. The cost for five nights was $228.45, with Wi-Fi.

Yuma has a population of 94,361 so there are many hotels/motels available. There was one my dentist recommended, the Q Casino. I checked it out on the way back from one of my appointments and it is very nice. At least the casino was well laid out; I didn't see any of the rooms.

Update: For my next trip I stayed at the Hotel Hacienda in town. It was only a few blocks from the dentist, had a pool, and allowed pets. They are owned by Sani Dental, they give you a break on your nightly rate.

What To Pack

Take whatever you normally would wear at a warm weather location. **And take cash.** Or at least get cash when you are in Yuma. Most dentists prefer cash. You can use credit cards, but check with them first. Offices charge a surcharge if you use a credit card.

There are several stores in Los Algodones. If you are looking for liquor, prescription drugs, or gifts, you're in luck. You can find those items everywhere. (*See picture of the drug menu board.*) A few stores also carry toiletries and food. If you cannot do without specific things like flavored potato chips or Mountain Dew, buy it in Yuma and carry it in yourself. You might be able to find what you want, but you don't want your trip to be spoiled because the stores didn't carry your favorite snack.

Prohibited Items

As stated above, you can take in packaged food, but do not bring in fresh fruit or vegetables. Other forbidden items are guns, bullets, explosives, recreational drugs. If you take prescription medicine, bring your prescription with you.

IV. THE TRIP

Los Algodones

So where is this dental mecca? It is a little town called Los Algodones (means "The Cotton"). It is the northernmost city in Mexico. It is only a 15 minute drive from Yuma, Arizona. If you want, you can stay in Yuma and cross over every day. That is what I did on my first trip. For my second trip I chose to stay in a hotel in the city. The hotel picked me up from the airport and the dental office was within walking distance I didn't need to rent a car.

Over a 10-year period the number of dentists has grown to over 350 all within ten minutes' walking distance from the U.S. border. On an average January day over 33,000 tourists walk across this international border.

Safety Issues

When I was there in 2010, I felt as safe as I do in Denver, Colorado, perhaps safer. There were armed guards at the border. I didn't see them going into Mexico; only upon leaving. I did some research and found postings from people who had been there in 2011. They said it was perfectly safe. Los Algodones is a small town filled with professionals so the drug cartels have left them alone. The only people I found that you had to pay attention to were the hawkers. They try to get you into their stores to buy something. There are also people who will try to talk you into going to another dentist.

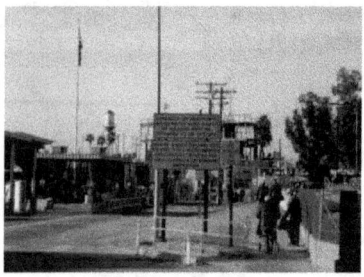

I took this before I saw the sign warning people not to take pictures of the border crossing. Ooops!

Los Algodones border

See the people on the right hand side of the picture? They are walking along a sidewalk, crossing the border into Los Algodones.

Update: For my next two trips, I stayed at the Hacienda in Mexico. It is very safe and they have a wall that surrounds the motel and an iron gate that is closed at night. I did hear about some people having problems in town after they visited a bar called the Green Door. I would caution against going out after night unless you are with a group of people.

Dentists, Optometrists & Drugstores

This next picture is my first view of the town itself. If you look closely, you will note there are seven signs for dentists. Pretty much the only businesses in Los Algodones are dentists, optometrists, liquor stores and pharmacies with a few restaurants thrown in to feed tourists.

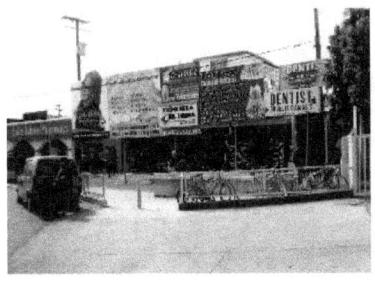

First view of Los Algodones

Los Algodones is a "medical city." Except for a few restaurants, bars and the numerous vendors who line the streets, there is nothing else there.

No movie theaters, no bowling alleys, no businesses in the way of recreation. The city holds events throughout the year. In January they hold drag races at the dunes. One time I was there in February and they had an outdoor concert with vendors selling food and trinkets. A Mexican Revolution Anniversary Parade is

17

held in November. In April there is an "Anniversary of Fish and Shrimp Taco."

I'm not sure what that is, but if you have a chance, eat at Fish and Shrimp Tacos. I had never had a fish taco I liked but I couldn't get enough of this place, along with everybody else. The line started at 10:30 and lasted throughout the afternoon.

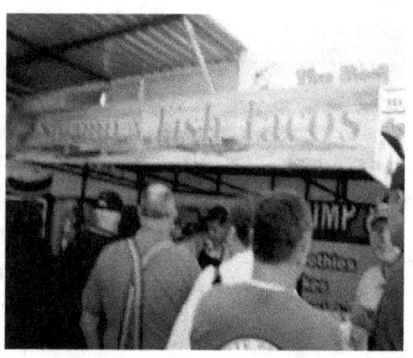

Don't worry, you can't miss this place. It is right across from a hyperbaric chamber. (*More about that later.*) Yes, a hyperbaric chamber, the kind that Michael Jackson used. The chamber that is used on scuba divers when they surface too fast and get the bends. The shop is right between a restaurant and a clothing store.

V. THE APPOINTMENT

Now that you know a little about Los Algodones, it's time for your appointment.

Dr. C. was on time and took me into his office. He was very good looking. Thank you, Tony! (Tony is my friend who recommended Dr. C.) His office looked like an American dentist office for the most part. He did have a spit sink *(something I have missed since they quit using them in the U.S.)*.

We talked for quite a while. He was very personable and friendly. I found out that Dr. C had worked in a dental office for several years in Oregon but had decided to return to Mexico to practice. He said he felt like patients in the U.S. were treated more like a number than a person. I told him that had been my experience in recent years.

One fun aspect of going to see Dr. C (when was the last time you had fun at a dentist office?) was right outside his office building was a restaurant with people eating and a band playing. While Dr. C talked to me, I could hear "By the Time I Get To Phoenix" by Glenn Campbell sung in Spanish. It was fun! Sure beats the piped music playing in U.S. dentist offices.

Dr. C took an X-ray and had the results 5 minutes later. When has that ever happened in a U.S. dental office? After looking at the X-ray, he decided he would feel more comfortable if his colleague, Dr. R. performed the root canal. Dr. R was located a few blocks away in Plaza Flamingo and Dr. C. walked me over there.

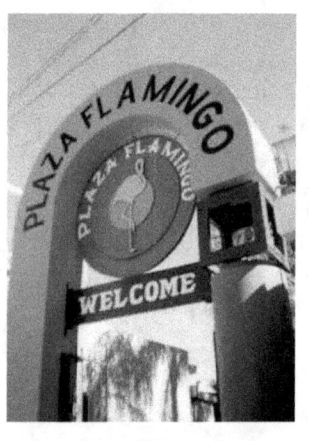

Dental Plaza

What service! In the outdoor patio area, there were tables set up for patients waiting to see the dentist. There were five dentists in this plaza.

Dr. R was in an office with his brother. There were two people in the waiting room when I arrived.

The only drawback to the whole dental trip is that sometimes you have to wait a long time. But remember, I didn't have an appointment with Dr. R. They thought they could get me in at noon, but it was 2:00 p.m. before I could be seen.

My wait was unlike any I have ever spent in a doctor's waiting room. There were six of us and we had a great time. Terry and Terry (husband and wife) were from Evergreen, Colorado and were traveling around the U.S. in their RV. There was another couple who came to Mexico every winter to see the dentist. There was a lady who had been coming down for several years. She told us that her daughter had MS and she brought her to Los Algodones for alternative health treatments she couldn't receive in the U.S. She said her daughter had used the hyperbaric chamber for some of her treatments.

Update: Now that I have been to Los Algodones several times, I have found that time is not as closely watched as here in the states. I quickly learned that if my appointment was at 2:00, I could leave my hotel at 2:00 and still have to wait a while. When you make you initial appointment, it would be wise to ask about wait times so you can plan accordingly. Of course, if there is a wait, there are plenty of vendors right outside the door to keep you amused for a long time.

Procedure

I waited a couple of hours and then April, the receptionist, told me Dr. R could see me. He took X-rays and within about two minutes, I was looking at the X-rays on a computer screen. The screen was attached to the arm of the light they pull down to see into your mouth. I have since talked to friends who have seen this type of X-ray procedure, but I had never seen it before. It was amazing! (*Since this trip I have seen dental offices in America have this equipment.*)

When Dr. R showed me the X-rays, he pointed out that my root canal had four roots instead of the usual three. When I returned home, I talked to a friend who is a dental hygienist. She said that was the sign of a good dentist because he noticed the fourth root. Sometimes it is not found and the patient has problems later.

Next came the Novocain. This is the part I always dread. It always has been extremely painful. *One time a U.S. dentist gave me a shot in the roof of my mouth and*

my eyes started uncontrollably darting
back and forth. It went on for a couple of
minute. It was extremely scary but the
doctor told me not to worry! Dr. R had me
move my lower jaw one way, my upper jaw
another and then gave me the shot. On a
scale of 1-10, with 10 being very painful, it
was less than a 1. **This alone was worth
the trip.**

He then put a rubber sheet across my
mouth and had just the tooth poke out
from the sheet. I had never had that done
before either. The sheet kept anything
from falling down my throat.

While he worked, there were two
assistants helping him. They were talking
through the whole procedure, but since
they were talking Spanish and I don't
know Spanish, I found it relaxing. It is a
pretty language. Don't worry, the dentists
all speak English so there is no
communication problem. When I left,
April gave me some antibiotics to take for
the next five days. No tequila for me!

This took place on Monday. I returned for
succeeding appointments with both Dr. C
and Dr. R throughout the week and all the
work was done on Thursday afternoon, as

promised. I was pleased with the work and with the professional demeanor of the dentists and staff. And of course, the cost for the work was great. The whole experience reminded me of my childhood dentist, Dr. Hale, and how going to the dentist doesn't have to be negative but can be an enjoyable experience.

VI. THE TOWN

I walked the whole town in about an hour. The shopping area is only four square blocks. There are a few houses, most of the homes are small, but there are a few mansions.

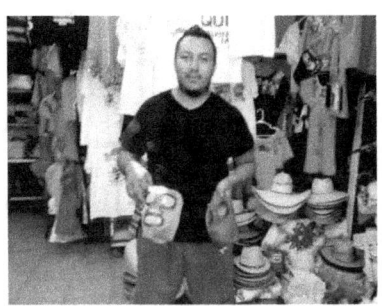

Bob the Vendor

My dentist at Oasis Dental used the crown making facility in town so it takes a fraction of the time to get crowns that it does in the U.S.

In addition to dentists, the main business of Los Algodones is street vendors. You can buy anything from clothes to jewelry to household goods. Keep in mind, most of the silver is low quality.

Update: There is a new industry blossoming in Los Algodones - holistic health. As mentioned before, there is a hyperbariac chamber.

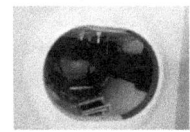

Hyperbaric Chamber

While there, I saw a naturopath. In his office, I saw a room where people were sitting in comfortable chairs with IVs running from their arms. They were getting heavy metals removed from their blood (chelation). A lot of people travel here for that purpose. There are many other methods of alternative health available here.

While waiting in line to go back across the border, I noticed a lot of people had bags of stuff they bought. It turned out, most of them were bringing back drugs.

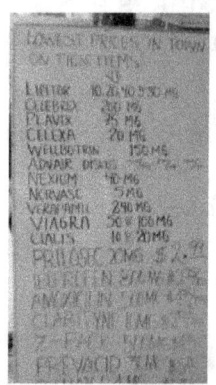

This sign was outside one pharmacies. They sell just about anything. If you buy brand name drugs, like Celebrex, you will pay the same price you do in the U.S. But if you buy generic, you will pay a fraction of the cost.

Friends placed orders with me so I bought 100 generic Claritin tabs for $2.98; 100 tabs of 800 mg Motrin for $2.75; and Prilosec for $2.99 (120 tabs). They make great Christmas presents. (*Just kidding.*)

VII. RECOMMENDATIONS

Dental Work

Do your homework before you go. Have a good idea of the work you want done before you get there. Dentistry is a cutthroat business down there. Dentists have representatives roaming the streets down there, trying to lure people into their office. Get different prices, by all means, but in the end, you have to feel comfortable with the dentist. My first appointment was with SaniDental but I switched to Oasis Dental. SaniDental has a reputation of pushing patients to get more work done than they actually need. Los Algodones is a small town and as such, the gossip flows freely. If you talk to the locals, you will find out all sorts of things. Of course, if the subject is dental work, the talk may just be to get you to come to a different dentist.

Dentists like cash so take cash with you. They do accept credit cards, but you will be charged a service fee.

Waiting times can vary but do not expect a 2:00 appointment to start right at 2:00.

Lodging

I have stayed in Yuma and Los Algodones. They both have their good points and drawbacks. Staying in Yuma means crossing the border every day. Going there is no problem, but if you park in the U.S. and come back from 2:00 to 5:00 p.m., the wait in line can be rather lengthy. This applies mainly from October to April. If you visit during the summer months, the wait is not as long.

I prefer staying in Los Algodones. There are a few places to stay; I stayed at The Hacienda. Each room was different and each one has WiFi and a small refrigerator.

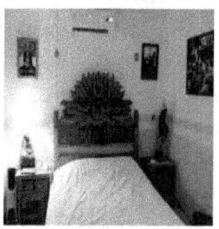

The Hacienda

There is an outdoor pool and a nice courtyard. SaniDental owns The Hacienda so if you have work done there, your room rate is reduced. Once I switched dentists, the room rate was $50 a night.

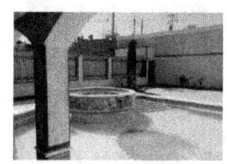

Pool at Hacienda

Dining

If you have a lot of
dental work done, you
may not be doing a lot
of eating. There are a
couple of grocery stores
in Los Algodones to buy
food. If you're lucky,
you'll be there on the
day they give away free
shots of tequila in the
grocery store!

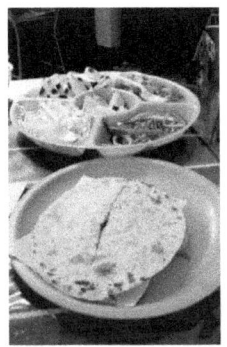

Quesadilla with
toppings

There are several restaurants to choose
from, the majority (if not all) serve Mexican
food. Be forewarned, the green chile is
much hotter than U.S. green chile. On the
whole, the food is very good. Some
restaurants have patios with bands
serenading the diners. The whole town is
a very festive place until around 5:00. AT
that time, the vendors close down and the
town rolls up the sidewalks.

VIII. LEAVING MEXICO

Remember, you need a passport to get back into the United States. It takes time for the agents to check everyone's passport so if you don't want to wait in line for hours, return before noon or after 5:00 p.m. *If you plan your trip during warm months, the waiting times can be shorter.* Otherwise, the wait can be extremely long. The best time to go to Mexico is June to September. From October to May is when the snowbirds flock there so wait times, both for appointments and returning to the U.S., are much longer. The first day I stood in line for two hours. There are benches to sit on along the way.

Even though the wait was long, there was plenty of entertainment to make the time pass quickly. It seemed that while one person was having work done, their spouse or friend was pounding down alcohol. We were treated to many drunk people singing, dancing, joking and basically having a good time.

Once you pass through the checkpoint, you walk a few yards and you are back across the U.S. border.

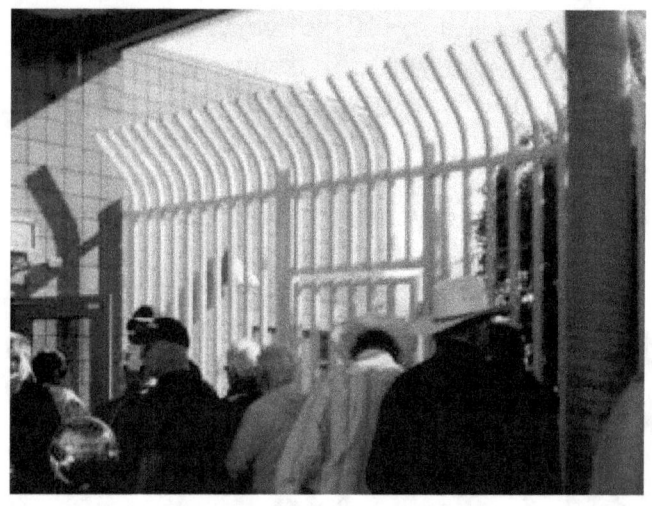

Returning to the U.S.

The border guards will check your bags. The laws on how many prescription drugs you can bring back is constantly changing, so before you go, find out the legal limit.

There are two secure parking lots where you can pay to park. If you drive across the border into Mexico, you have to get car insurance. It's the law.

IX. TOTAL COST

This is what I paid for my first dental trip to Los Algodones in 2010. I have since returned because of the great prices and the dentists are qualified, very personable and friendly.

> $682.00 - Airfare, rental car, hotel, gas, food
> $200.00 - Root canal
> $180.00 - Porcelain crown
> $ 20.00 - X-rays
> $ 80.00 - Fillings

$1,152.00 - Less than a $1200 root canal in the U.S. Dr. C also built up one of my teeth and charged $40.00. In the U.S. it would have cost another $150.00

Pre-Travel Points To Remember

- ✓ Establish contact with the dentist before traveling to Mexico.
- ✓ Have an idea of the type of work you need done.
- ✓ Check to see if the dentist has Skype. That way you could talk to them

- ✓ directly. If you both have a web cam, you can see each other.
- ✓ Make sure you feel comfortable with the dentist. If you don't feel
- ✓ comfortable with them, find another.
- ✓ Allow up to 6 weeks to receive your passport.
- ✓ Take cash or bank card so you can get cash in Yuma.
- ✓ If you plan on driving into Mexico, obtain car insurance before you go. Easiest way to do this is purchase it online.
- ✓ If you need a plane ticket, Tuesday is the best day to purchase it.

X. CONCLUSION

Would I do it again? You bet! And I have.
The excellent service, the feeling that you
are a person, not a number, it's an
adventure, great prices - I don't see a
down side. Overall, it was a great
experience. The majority of people you see
and meet are Americans and Canadians.
And everyone is in a festive mood.

Keep in mind why you are there. You are
getting dental work done. No matter how
great the service is, it's tiring and not fun
having your teeth worked on. So don't
plan on partying. Plus, you may have to
take antibiotics. I found that after my
appointments, I usually went back to the
hotel and stayed there.

Thank you for reading my book. I hope it
calmed your fears about having dental
work done in Mexico. If you enjoyed it,
won't you please take a moment to leave a
review at your favorite book retailer?
Thank you.

Ellen

About the Author

Ellen L. Hughes founded The McKee Company in 1994. The goal was to make life easier for people with products that build confidence in specific areas and life events. Whether in the form of a book, software or other type of medium, the focus is always to give you the means to find what you need, easily and quickly.

The first project was to organize government auctions. We researched government agencies that sold surplus property and organized the information, creating the Government Auctions/Sales Manual. *Reader's Digest, Kiplinger, Bottom Line/Personal, Worth* and several other national and trade magazines endorsed it.

The second project was to create a tool (Office Wizard) to help business owners easily organize their businesses so they could turn their attention to growing their companies.

After that came Adventures With Natural Healing, Be A Smart Client and many other books that can be found at www.TheMcKeeCompany.com

Other titles by Ellen L. Hughes

105 Ways to Make Money at Home

Adventures With Natural Healing - *A Health Junkie's Journey Through Alternative Medicine*

Be A Smart Client - *How To Hire The Best Lawyer and Help Win Your Case*

Dental Heaven - *Get A Great Smile Without Paying Through The Nose*

Government Auctions/Sales Manual

Home Office Handbook

Re-Energize Yourself - *Simple Techniques to Recharge Your Body and Mind*

Office Wizard - *A Personalized Office Procedures Manual (software)*

More to come…

If you have a suggestion for a book, please contact Hughes.